EMBRACING VEGANISM

A COMPREHENSIVE GUIDE TO PLANT BASED LIVING

A.D RAMS

Contents

CHAPTER ONE

Introduction

A growing number of people are adopting veganism as a way of life and diet due to ethical, environmental, and health reasons. Essentially, veganism is the practice of not using any animal products for clothing, food, or other purposes. This entails cutting off animal-derived foods and beverages from one's diet and way of life, such as meat, poultry, fish, dairy, eggs, and honey.

The three main tenets of veganism are personal wellness, environmental sustainability, and compassion for animals. Due to ethical concerns about animal welfare and the abuse of animals in the food business, a large number of vegans opt to eschew animal products. Vegans want to minimize the exploitation of animals for human use and to decrease the need for animal agriculture by switching to a plant-based diet.

Environmental reasons are a driving force behind veganism in addition to ethical ones. Deforestation, water pollution, greenhouse gas emissions, and other environmental problems are all significantly impacted by animal husbandry. Vegans try to lessen their environmental impact and their carbon footprint by consuming more plant-based foods than animal products.

Many possible health benefits of veganism have been linked to the lifestyle. When compared to a standard omnivorous diet, a well-planned vegan diet can be lower in saturated fat and cholesterol and higher in vitamins, minerals, fiber, and antioxidants. A plant-based diet has been linked to a decreased risk of heart disease, type 2 diabetes, and some types of cancer, among other chronic conditions.

A vegan lifestyle is now more accessible than ever because to the large growth in vegan-friendly materials and products available in recent years. For individuals interested in making the switch to veganism, there are plenty of resources and support networks accessible, including plant-based meat substitutes, dairy-free goods, vegan cookbooks, and online groups.

All things considered, becoming vegan is a deliberate decision to live a life that is consistent with compassion, sustainability, and health. Whether driven by an interest in protecting animals, the environment, or one's own health, vegans are a part of an expanding movement that aims to create a world that is more moral, sustainable, and compassionate.

The definition and tenets of veganism

Veganism is a philosophy and way of life that emphasizes not using any animal products for clothing, food, or other purposes. Fundamentally, health, environmental, and ethical concerns are what motivate veganism.

The compassion for animals is at the core of the vegan worldview. Because they are concerned about how animals are treated and exploited in sectors like factory farming, animal testing, and entertainment, vegans opt not to consume animal products. Vegans aim to reduce their involvement in animal suffering and exploitation by avoiding meat, dairy, eggs, honey, and other goods derived from animals.

Environmental reasons are a driving force behind veganism in addition to ethical ones. Deforestation, greenhouse gas emissions, water pollution, and other environmental problems are significantly exacerbated by animal agriculture. Choosing plant-based diets over animal products is how vegans want to lessen their impact on the environment and encourage sustainability.

There are a lot of possible health benefits linked with being vegan. Rich in fruits, vegetables, whole grains, legumes, nuts, and seeds, a well-planned vegan diet can supply vital elements including antioxidants, fiber, vitamins, and minerals. A plant-based diet has been linked to a decreased risk of heart disease, type 2 diabetes, and some types of cancer, among other chronic conditions.

All things considered, going vegan is a deliberate decision to live a life that is consistent with compassion, environmental responsibility, and individual health. It is a way of living that aims to lessen damage to animals, lessen the influence on the environment, and enhance the wellbeing of both people and the earth. Vegans work to make the world a more moral, ecological, and compassionate place for all living things through their dietary and lifestyle choices.

Veganism's Historical Context and Evolution

The idea of avoiding animal products has been around for centuries and is rooted in a number of philosophical, theological, and cultural traditions. But the vegan movement as we know it now began in the middle of the 20th century and has changed dramatically since then. Here is a quick synopsis of the background and development of veganism:

Ancient Influences: For ethical, religious, or health-related reasons, some people and cultures have abstained from eating some animal products or have adopted vegetarianism throughout history. For instance, ancient Greek and Indian philosophers supported vegetarian diets, and some religious traditions like Buddhism and Jainism promote the values of non-violence and animal compassion.

Early Advocacy: Throughout the 18th and 19th centuries, a number of people and groups started promoting animal rights and vegetarianism in Western societies. Prominent figures like Percy Bysshe Shelley, Henry Salt, and John Wesley advocated for compassionate treatment of animals and ethical vegetarianism.

Creation of Veganism: In 1944, Donald Watson and a group of British friends who shared his views founded the Vegan Society, coining the term "vegan". They used the phrase to set themselves apart from other vegetarians who ate eggs and dairy products. A vegan lifestyle is one that aims to abstain from all animal exploitation and abuse.

Expansion and Recognition: Over the ensuing decades, veganism gained popularity and traveled outside of the UK to other countries. The Vegan Society persisted in advancing veganism by writings, events, and lobbying. Growing numbers of people are realizing that veganism is a unique way of living based on moral values and animal care.

Mainstream Awareness: The popularity and awareness of veganism have skyrocketed in recent years. The vegan movement has grown as a result of various factors, including personal health, environmental sustainability, and animal welfare issues. Growing knowledge of veganism and its advantages has also been aided by the emergence of social media, documentaries, and celebrity endorsements.

Product Diversification: As veganism gains popularity, more plant-based food options, cruelty-free cosmetics, vegan clothing, and other vegan-friendly products are becoming available. Businesses have expanded their selection of vegan substitutes for conventional animal-based items in response to consumer demand.

Global Movement: With a broad network of people supporting human health, environmental sustainability, and animal rights, veganism is now acknowledged as a global movement. Vegan groups, activities, and campaigns never stop highlighting the advantages of veganism and advancing the cause of a more sympathetic and sustainable world for all living things.

In general, the historical development of veganism is indicative of an increasing concern for environmental sustainability, animal welfare, and individual health. With veganism gaining popularity, it is becoming a more influential force for good, encouraging people to lead more sustainable and compassionate lives.

Goals and Intentions behind Becoming a Vegan

Although the motivations behind and goals of a vegan lifestyle can differ from person to person, they frequently include ethical, environmental, and health-related factors. The following are some typical goals and motives for adopting veganism:

Ethical Considerations: Concern for animal welfare is a common reason for vegan lifestyle adoption. Vegans try to limit their involvement in animal suffering and exploitation in sectors including factory farming, animal testing, and entertainment by giving up meat, dairy, eggs, honey, and other goods derived from animals. Living in accordance with the ideals of kindness, nonviolence, and respect for all living things is the main goal.

Environmental Sustainability: Environmental issues are a common driving force behind veganism. Deforestation, greenhouse gas emissions, water pollution, and habitat devastation are all directly related to animal agriculture. Choosing plant-based diets over animal products is how vegans want to lessen their impact on the environment and encourage sustainability. Reducing the influence on the environment and protecting natural resources for next generations are the goals.

Health and Well-Being: There are a lot of possible health advantages to switching to a vegan lifestyle.

CHAPTER TWO

Rich in fruits, vegetables, whole grains, legumes, nuts, and seeds, a well-planned vegan diet can supply vital elements including antioxidants, fiber, vitamins, and minerals. A plant-based diet has been linked to a decreased risk of heart disease, type 2 diabetes, and some types of cancer, among other chronic conditions. The aim is to enhance individual health and wellness through the selection of wholesome, plant-based diets.

Social Justice and Equity: Global injustice, human rights, and food justice are only a few of the larger social justice issues that veganism is linked to. Vegans seek to solve challenges including food insecurity, access to nutrient-dense foods, and healthcare inequities by promoting plant-based diets and sustainable food systems. Promoting social justice, equity, and inclusivity within communities and food systems is the goal.

Spiritual and Cultural Values: Compassion, non-violence, and respect for life are some of the spiritual or cultural ideas that some people feel have an impact on their decision to embrace a vegan lifestyle. Veganism may be in line with the teachings of religious traditions that support respect for all living things and ahimsa (non-harming), including Buddhism, Jainism, and some branches of Hinduism. Living in accordance with spiritual or cultural ideals and values is the goal.

All things considered, there are many different and related reasons to embrace a vegan lifestyle, including ethical, environmental, health, social, and cultural factors. By adopting a vegan lifestyle, people aim to improve their own health and wellbeing as well as the compassionate, sustainable, and egalitarian environment they live in for all living things.

Comprehending the Nutrition of Vegans

Comprehending vegan nutrition is crucial to guaranteeing that persons who adopt a plant-based lifestyle fulfill their nutritional requirements and sustain ideal wellness. The following are important vegan dietary considerations:

Plant-Based Protein Sources: Protein is a necessary macronutrient that aids in immunological response, hormone production, tissue growth, and repair. Although most people identify protein with animal products, there are many of plant-based protein sources that can satisfy dietary requirements. They include specific grains like amaranth and buckwheat, as well as beans, lentils, chickpeas, tofu, tempeh, seitan, edamame, and quinoa. You can make sure you're getting enough protein by eating a range of these plant-based protein sources throughout the day.

Foods High in Calcium: Calcium is necessary for healthy teeth and bones, as well as for muscle and nerve function. Although dairy products are the conventional source of calcium, there are a variety of plant-based substitutes that can be used instead, such as calcium-set tofu, fortified juices, plant milks (like soy, almond, or oat milk), leafy green vegetables (like bok choy, collard greens, and kale), almonds, tahini, and tofu that has been fortified with calcium sulfate.

Iron Absorption: Red blood cell production and oxygen transportation throughout the body depend on iron. Legumes, lentils, tofu, tempeh, soybeans, spinach, kale, swiss chard, fortified cereals, quinoa, pumpkin seeds, and sesame seeds are plant-based sources of iron.

Consuming iron-rich foods with foods high in vitamin C, such as citrus fruits, berries, bell peppers, tomatoes, and broccoli, can improve the absorption of iron.

Vitamin B12 Supplementation: Red blood cell production, DNA synthesis, and neuron function all depend on vitamin B12. Since animal products contain the majority of vitamin B12, vegans must get their fill from supplements or fortified foods such plant milks, cereals for breakfast, nutritional yeast, and meat alternatives. It is advised to regularly consume foods fortified with B12 or take a B12 supplement to guarantee an appropriate intake.

Omega-3 Fatty Acids: These important fats are involved in brain development, heart health, and the control of inflammation. Omega-3s are commonly found in fatty fish, but vegans can also get them from plant-based foods including flaxseeds, chia seeds, hemp seeds, walnuts, and algae-based supplements (which contain the active forms of omega-3s, EPA and DHA).

Balanced Meals and Snacks: The key to achieving a vegan diet's nutrient requirements is consuming a range of entire plant foods, such as fruits, vegetables, whole grains, legumes, nuts, and seeds. To guarantee a wide range of nutrients, try to incorporate different colors, textures, and flavors into your meals and snacks. Pay attention to serving sizes and arrange meals high in fiber, protein, healthy fats, and carbs on your plate in a balanced manner.

See a certified Dietitian: If you're new to veganism or have particular health issues, you might want to see a plant-based nutrition specialist certified dietitian. A dietician may assist with evaluating your nutritional needs, making tailored suggestions, and making sure that you're getting enough nutrients on a vegan diet.

People can live on a vegan diet while promoting their general health and well-being by emphasizing nutrient-rich whole foods, including a range of plant-based protein sources, and paying attention to important nutrients like calcium, iron, vitamin B12, and omega-3 fatty acids.

Numerous possible health benefits of veganism have been linked to it, with both empirical and research data supporting this claim. The following health benefits of living a vegan lifestyle have been demonstrated, though individual experiences may differ:

Heart Health: Studies have shown a lower risk of heart disease in people who follow a plant-based diet high in fruits, vegetables, whole grains, legumes, nuts, and seeds. Because vegan diets often contain less cholesterol and saturated fat, they may help lower blood cholesterol levels and reduce the risk of heart disease and stroke. Additionally, by lowering blood pressure and raising cholesterol, the high fiber content of plant-based diets can support heart health.

Weight management: Compared to omnivorous diets, vegan diets are frequently higher in fiber and lower in calories, which may help with weight loss and maintenance. Plant-based diets typically contain more nutrients and less calories, which helps people feel satisfied for longer periods of time and consume fewer calories overall. Research indicates that as compared to non-vegans, vegans typically have lower body mass indices (BMIs) and lower rates of obesity.

Decreased Risk of Type 2 Diabetes: Plant-based diets have the potential to enhance glycemic control in diabetics and reduce the risk of acquiring type 2 diabetes. Plant-based diets have a high fiber content and a low glycemic index, which can help control blood sugar levels and enhance insulin sensitivity. Studies indicate that vegan diets may be especially helpful in managing and preventing type 2 diabetes.

Reduced Cancer Risk: Research has linked eating a diet high in fruits, vegetables, and other plant-based foods to a lower risk of developing several types of cancer. Antioxidants, vitamins, minerals, and phytochemicals included in vegan diets are generally abundant and have the potential to prevent the development of cancer. Research indicates that there could be a difference in the incidence of breast, prostate, and colon cancer between vegans and non-vegans.

Better Digestive Health: Diets rich in plants naturally include a lot of fiber, which helps to keep the gut flora balanced, encourage regular bowel movements, and prevent constipation. Additionally, eating a diet high in fiber lowers the chance of developing digestive diseases like diverticulitis, hemorrhoids, and irritable bowel syndrome (IBS). Prebiotics, which enhance overall digestive wellbeing by nourishing good gut flora, can be obtained through consuming a variety of plant-based meals.

Lower Risk of Chronic Disease: Studies have linked vegan diets to a lower risk of metabolic syndrome, hypertension, and hyperlipidemia, among other chronic diseases. Vegans enjoy a diet naturally rich in vitamins, minerals, antioxidants, and phytochemicals that support general health and reduce inflammation by focusing on whole, minimally processed plant foods. It has been demonstrated that plant-based diets reduce oxidative stress and inflammatory indicators, which are linked to the emergence of chronic diseases.

lifetime and Longevity: Research indicates that adopting a vegan diet may lead to a longer lifetime and lower risks of death from specific illnesses. Vegan diets may increase overall longevity and quality of life in later years by lowering the risk of chronic diseases, increasing heart health, and helping people maintain a healthy weight.

Although switching to a vegan lifestyle can have many positive effects on health, it's crucial to remember that each person's results may differ depending on a variety of factors, including lifestyle choices, genetic makeup, past medical history, and the quality of their general diet. A well-balanced vegan diet that tackles any nutrient shortages and meets dietary demands is also crucial. Examples of these include vitamin B12, iron, calcium, omega-3 fatty acids, and vitamin D. It is possible to make sure that you are fulfilling your dietary needs and maintaining your general health while following a vegan diet by speaking with a licensed dietitian or other healthcare professional.

Environmental and Ethical Considerations

Adopting a vegan lifestyle is frequently driven by ethical and environmental concerns in addition to its health benefits. Here is a closer examination of these crucial elements:

Moral Aspects to Take into Account:

Animal Welfare: Concern for the welfare of animals is one of the main moral justifications for veganism. Because they disagree with how animals are treated in businesses like factory farming, dairy production, egg production, and animal experimentation, many people opt to forgo consuming animal products. Due to frequent practices in these industries, including confinement, overcrowding, mutilations, and harsh methods of slaughter, vegans reject the use of animal products on moral grounds.

Compassion and Non-Violence: The core values of veganism are respect for all living things, compassion, and non-violence. Supporters contend that every animal, regardless of species, has a right to exist unharmed and unexploited. Vegans seek to reduce their own animal suffering and to encourage a more moral and compassionate attitude toward food and lifestyle choices by refraining from using animal products.

CHAPTER THREE

Environmental Factors to Be Considered

Climate Change: Deforestation, water pollution, greenhouse gas emissions, and habitat degradation are all significantly impacted by animal husbandry. Methane is a powerful greenhouse gas that is produced by livestock production, which includes raising cattle, pigs, and poultry. This gas contributes to climate change. Vegans seek to lessen the environmental impact of food production and reduce their carbon footprint by cutting back on or giving up the consumption of animal products.

Resource conservation: A lot of land, water, and energy are needed for animal husbandry. Raising cattle, processing meat, dairy, and eggs, and growing feed crops for them all use a lot of resources and worsen pollution, water scarcity, and land degradation. Diets based primarily on plants are more resource-efficient since they require less energy, water, and land to produce food, protecting the environment and fostering sustainability.

Preservation of Biodiversity: The health of ecosystems and biodiversity are threatened by deforestation caused by livestock grazing and feed crop cultivation. Forest clearing for agriculture causes habitat destruction, wildlife displacement, and the extinction of certain species. Vegans promote the preservation of natural ecosystems, biodiversity, and ecosystem integrity by moving away from animal agriculture and in favor of plant-based food systems.

Ultimately, the vegan movement is centered on ethical and environmental issues, encouraging people to make decisions that are consistent with the values of compassion, non-violence, sustainability, and respect for the environment. A vegan lifestyle can help people promote environmental stewardship, address global issues like climate change, deforestation, and biodiversity loss, and create a more moral, sustainable, and compassionate world for all living things.

Making the Switch to a Vegan Lifestyle

Making the switch to a vegan lifestyle can be a fulfilling journey that supports moral, environmental, and health objectives. The following advice will help to ensure a more seamless and sustainable transition:

Educate Yourself: Invest some time in learning about the ethical, environmental, and health consequences of veganism. Knowing why you choose to adopt a vegan diet will inspire and strengthen your resolve to stick with the new way of living.

Take It Slowly: Adopting a vegan lifestyle doesn't have to happen all at once. Think on progressively consuming fewer animal products and consuming more plant-based foods. Increase the amount of fruits, veggies, whole grains, legumes, nuts, and seeds you eat, and then progressively cut out animal products over time.

Try New Plant-Based Recipes , Ingredients and Substitutes: Experiment with Plant-Based Foods. To find different flavors and textures, try experimenting with tofu, tempeh, seitan, lentils, beans, and a range of fruits, vegetables, grains, and nuts. In the kitchen, use your imagination and enjoy experimenting with plant-based baking and cooking.

Look for Vegan Substitutes: Swap out your favorite animal-based products for vegan ones. These days, there are a lot of plant-based substitutes for items originating from animals, such as dairy, eggs, cheese, milk, yogurt, and meat. Shop online, at restaurants, and at grocery stores for vegan versions of your favorite dishes.

Read Labels: Develop the practice of reading ingredient lists and labels to spot components derived from animals in packaged goods. Keep an eye out for commonly used animal products including casein, whey, gelatin, honey, and some food colorings (like carmine). To make educated decisions, familiarize yourself with labels and certifications that are vegan-friendly.

Plan and Prepare Meals: Following a vegan diet can be easier if meals are planned and prepared in advance. Every week, set aside time to organize your meals, create a shopping list, and prepare items ahead of time. You can save time and make sure you always have wholesome, plant-based meals available by batch cooking and meal planning.

Seek Support: To get inspiration, motivation, and support, get in touch with fellow vegans. Participate in local meetup groups, online forums, social media groups, and vegan communities to ask questions, exchange experiences, and gain knowledge from like-minded individuals. Being around by people who share your values might help you overcome obstacles and maintain motivation.

Be Kind and Flexible with Yourself: Keep in mind that adopting a vegan diet is a personal journey that you are free to go at your own speed. Try to be gentle with yourself and give yourself some leeway while you make the adjustment. Prioritize progress above perfection, and acknowledge and appreciate your accomplishments along the way.

Remain Knowledgeable and Receptive: Educate yourself about the diet, preparation methods, and lifestyle advice for vegans. Continue to be receptive to new cuisines and vegan lifestyle ideas. Keep learning about the advantages of veganism and the ways you can make the world a more compassionate and sustainable place.

You may make the process of switching to a vegan lifestyle more bearable and pleasurable by proceeding cautiously and gradually. Keep in mind that each step you take toward being a vegan is a step in the right direction toward living out your principles and improving the welfare of animals, the environment, and your own health.

Recipes and Meal Planning for Vegans

Making the switch to a vegan lifestyle requires meal preparation and experimentation with new dishes to make sure you're consuming a healthy, balanced diet. To get you started, consider these vegan-friendly recipes and meal planning advice:

For breakfast:

Vegan Pancakes: To create the batter, combine flour, baking powder, a little amount of salt, and plant-based milk (such soy or almond). Cook till golden brown on a nonstick pan. Garnish with chopped nuts, fresh fruit, and maple syrup.

Avocado Toast: Spread sliced tomatoes, mashed avocado, and a sprinkle of olive oil, salt, and pepper on top of toast made with whole-grain bread. For added taste, you can top with sliced radishes, sprouts, or a sprinkling of nutritional yeast.

Blend frozen bananas, berries, spinach, and plant-based milk in a smoothie bowl until smooth. For a filling and healthy breakfast, transfer into a bowl and garnish with granola, sliced fruit, shredded coconut, and a dollop of nut butter.

Lunch:

Veggie Wrap: Stuff bell peppers, avocado slices, shredded carrots, cucumber slices, spinach leaves, and hummus into a whole-grain tortilla. For a convenient and wholesome lunch, roll it firmly and cut into pinwheels.

Quinoa salad: Prepare the quinoa per the directions on the package, then set aside to cool. Add green beans, corn, cucumber, red onion, cherry tomatoes, sliced bell peppers, and a vinaigrette consisting of lemon juice, olive oil, garlic, and herbs. Serve cold for a light and high-protein lunch.

Bake sweet potatoes until they are soft, then cut them open and stuff them with a mixture of chopped cilantro, sliced avocado, black beans, and salsa. Add a lime wedge and a dollop of cashew cream or dairy-free yogurt on top.

Vegetable Stir-Fry: In a skillet with garlic, ginger, and soy sauce, sauté cubed tofu, broccoli florets, bell peppers, snap peas, carrots, and mushrooms. Serve with quinoa or brown rice for an easy and filling supper.

Chickpea Curry: In a pot, sauté onions, garlic, and spices (such turmeric, cumin, and curry powder) until aromatic. Add the diced tomatoes, spinach, coconut milk, and canned chickpeas. Simmer until thoroughly cooked, then serve with naan bread or over rice.

Make Vegan Pasta Primavera by following the directions on the package for whole-grain pasta. Garlic, herbs, olive oil, and sautéed zucchini, yellow squash, cherry tomatoes, and asparagus. For a tasty and light pasta dish, toss with cooked spaghetti, lemon zest, fresh basil, and a dash of nutritional yeast.

Munchies:

Fresh Fruit: For a light and revitalizing snack, savor a choice of fresh fruits, including apples, bananas, oranges, berries, and grapes.

Carrots, celery, bell peppers, and cucumbers should all be sliced up and served with a side of hummus for dipping.

Trail Mix: For a filling and energizing on-the-go snack, combine nuts, seeds, dried fruit, and dark chocolate chips.

Tips for Meal Planning:

Make a plan: Set aside some time each week to organize your snacks and meals. Make a list of the products you'll need for your shopping trip and search for vegan recipes online or in cookbooks.

Batch Cooking: Make big quantities of grains, beans, and roasted veggies in advance to use for several meals over the week. Meal prep can be streamlined and time-saving using this.

Maintain Balance: To make sure you're eating a well-rounded and balanced diet, try to eat a range of foods from all dietary groups, such as fruits, vegetables, whole grains, legumes, nuts, and seeds.

Be Adaptable: Don't be scared to try out novel flavors and ingredients. Using imagination and experimenting is key to vegan cooking.

You may have a tasty and nourishing vegan diet that promotes your health and well-being by planning ahead and including a range of plant-based foods into your meals and snacks.

Advice for Meal Planning and Grocery Shopping

Changing to a vegan diet requires a few tweaks to your weekly grocery shopping and meal planning schedule. The following advice will assist you in navigating the process:

Purchasing groceries:

Plan Ahead: Spend some time creating a shopping list and organizing your weekly menu before you go to the store. This will guarantee that you have all the components you need and help you keep organized.

Read Labels: Develop the practice of reading ingredient lists and labels to spot components derived from animals in packaged goods. Be wary of common animal additives like honey, whey, casein, gelatin, and some food colorings. Become familiar with certifications and labeling that are suitable for vegans.

Investigate New Foods: Use this chance to investigate foods and ingredients that you may not have previously tried. Try a variety of fruits, veggies, whole grains, legumes, nuts, seeds, and plant-based substitutes for dairy, meat, and eggs.

Stock Up on Staples: Make sure your pantry is well-stocked with basic foods like rice, quinoa, pasta, canned beans, lentils, and tomatoes, as well as nuts, seeds, and nut butter, as well as seasonings, herbs, and sauces. Several vegan dishes can be built around these adaptable ingredients.

Shop the Periphery: Concentrate on your grocery store shopping around the perimeter, where you'll discover plant-based substitutes, fresh produce, grains, legumes, nuts, and seeds. Restrict your intake of packaged and processed foods from the center aisles.

Purchase in quantity: To save money and cut down on packaging waste, think about purchasing some things in quantity. Find bulk bins or purchase more of the grains, beans, nuts, and seeds you frequently use.

Encourage Local Farmers Markets: For fresh, in-season vegetables and locally sourced goods, visit your local farmers market or cooperative. Purchasing locally can help local small-scale farmers and lessen your influence on the environment.

Preparing Meals:

Prepare Ahead: Schedule a weekly period for meal preparation and large-scale cooking. To save time during the week, chop veggies, cook grains and beans, and make sauces and dressings ahead of time.

Plan for Leftovers: Make bigger dinner quantities and make a conscious effort to have leftovers. You can make fresh dishes out of leftovers or have simple lunches or dinners all week long.

Utilize Time-Saving Appliances: To expedite food preparation, make an investment in time-saving appliances like a pressure cooker, slow cooker, or instant pot. These equipment can greatly simplify and speed up the process of cooking grains, beans, and soups.

Keep It Simple: You don't have to prepare extravagant dinners every single day. Put an emphasis on healthy, straightforward recipes that call for few ingredients and little time to prepare. A lot of vegan dishes may be prepared in under 30 minutes.

Be Creative: Don't be scared to use your imagination in the kitchen and try out various flavors, textures, and culinary traditions. Enjoy experimenting with new recipes, making beloved dishes vegan, and learning more about the wonderful world of plant-based cooking.

Keep Your Kitchen Organized: Make sure your kitchen is well-stocked with necessary tools and supplies. To make meal preparation easier, buy high-quality knives, cutting boards, pots, and pans. You should also maintain a clean, organized pantry and refrigerator.

You can ease into a more comfortable and seamless transition to a vegan lifestyle by being organized, making advance plans, and shopping wisely. Try out new meals and ideas, and don't be afraid to ask for assistance or use internet resources such as blogs and vegan cookbooks for inspiration. You will eventually create your own habits and preferences that serve your moral principles, environmental objectives, and well-being.

Social Situations and Eating Out

With a little preparation and communication, navigating social events and eating out as a vegan can be delightful and manageable. Here are some pointers for vegans looking to socialize and eat out:

Eating Outside:

Do Your Research: Look up a restaurant's menu online or give them a call to find out if they provide vegan options before making a decision. Nowadays, a lot of eateries can fulfill special dietary requirements or provide vegan-friendly menu items.

Selecting Vegan-Friendly Restaurants: Seek out eateries with a range of vegetarian and vegan options, or those that specialize in vegan or plant-based food. Vegan-friendly cuisine can be found frequently in ethnic restaurants like Thai, Indian, Mexican, and Middle Eastern ones.

Communicate Your Needs: When placing an order, don't be afraid to let the waitress know that you follow a vegan diet and request that certain meals be made vegan-friendly. The majority of eateries are flexible with regard to dietary requirements and preferences.

Be Adaptable: Although it's wonderful to discover eateries that cater specifically to vegans, be ready to adjust or substitute menu items as needed. For instance, you can request that dishes be prepared without cheese or beef, or that more tofu or vegetables be included.

Search for Hidden Ingredients: Keep an eye out for any unidentified animal ingredients in dressings, garnishes, broths, and sauces. If you're unsure, find out about ingredients or possible cross-contamination.

CHAPTER FOUR

Be Thankful and Civil: Express gratitude to staff members who accommodate your dietary restrictions as well as to eateries that provide vegan options. A good mood and courteous conversation go a long way toward guaranteeing a satisfying eating experience.

Social Contexts:

Communicate in Advance: If you're going to a social event or gathering where food will be provided, you might want to let the host know ahead of time about any dietary restrictions you may have. Offer to bring a dish to share that is vegan or make suggestions for vegan-friendly menu items.

Give Advice: If you're having a potluck or dining at a friend's house, give advice on vegan-friendly recipes that the whole group will like. Give recipes or advice on vegan substitutes and ingredients.

Always bring vegan snacks with you to social events or get-togethers, especially if you're not sure what kind of food will be available. By doing this, you may be sure that you'll have something to eat and avoid feeling lonely or hungry.

Be Ready to Educate: There may be individuals who are unsure or inquisitive about veganism. Make sure you are ready to respond positively and without passing judgment when people ask about your lifestyle and food choices. Take use of the chance to inform and motivate them to adopt a vegan diet.

Keep Your Attention on the Company: Keep in mind that the purpose of social gatherings is to make new friends and enjoy each other's company. Pay attention to the food, but also to the conversation, laughing, and shared experiences.

Examine Vegan-Friendly Activities: If you're looking for ways to spend time with friends and family that are friendly to veganism, think about planning picnics, cooking workshops, potlucks, or trips to vegan eateries. This lets you discover vegan food and connect over similar passions and life experiences.

You can confidently manage eating out and social situations as a vegan by being prepared, articulating your needs, being adaptable, and keeping a happy attitude. Regardless of dietary restrictions, always remember to have fun and concentrate on the relationships you form with others.

Beyond Food Veganism

Beyond nutrition decisions, veganism touches on many facets of daily living, such as clothing, personal care products, home goods, and ethical issues. Here are some ideas for extending veganism outside of food:

Items for Personal Care:

Examine Labels: On personal care items including skincare, makeup, shampoo, conditioner, soap, and toothpaste, look for labels certifying the product is cruelty-free and vegan-friendly. Steer clear of goods that include substances like carmine, beeswax, and lanolin that are sourced from animals.

Select Vegan substitutes: Go for plant-based moisturizers, mineral cosmetics, and cruelty-free skincare brands as vegan substitutes for popular personal care items. These days, a lot of businesses provide vegan solutions devoid of products originating from animals and animal experimentation.

Homemade Remedies: Take into consideration creating your own natural personal care products at home with components like shea butter, coconut oil, essential oils, and plant extracts. Online recipes abound for making your own DIY hygiene, haircare, and skincare items.

Outfits and Accessory Items:

Shop Ethically: Select apparel and accessories from materials like cotton, hemp, bamboo, linen, synthetic leather, and microfiber that are suitable for vegans. Steer clear of materials like down, leather, fur, silk, and wool that come from animals.

Support Vegan Brands: Seek out clothing companies that place a high value on sustainable and ethical practices, such as the use of vegan materials, fair labor standards, and environmentally friendly production techniques. Many businesses now provide fashionable lines of shoes, purses, accessories, and apparel that are cruelty-free.

Secondhand and Thrifting: If you're looking for gently used apparel and accessories, check out thrift stores, consignment stores, and online resale marketplaces. Purchasing used goods lowers waste and the need for newly manufactured goods generated from animals.

Domestic Goods:

Select Cruelty-Free: Seek for home goods that don't include animal testing, such as dish soap, cleaning supplies, laundry detergent, and air fresheners. Many businesses provide plant-based, vegan products that are cruelty-free and tested on animals.

Handmade Cleaners: Using basic components like vinegar, baking soda, lemon juice, and essential oils, create your own environmentally friendly cleaning solutions. Homemade cleaning solutions are safe, economical, and devoid of dangerous chemicals that are present in store-bought cleaning supplies.

Moral Aspects to Take into Account:

Animal Advocacy: Take part in animal advocacy and provide your support to groups that defend animals and advance veganism. Advocate for animal rights in your town, take part in advocacy activities, and volunteer at animal shelters.

Environmental Awareness: Acknowledge how animal agriculture affects the environment and back programs that encourage conservation and sustainability. Participate in eco-friendly activities, join environmental organizations, and inform others about the relationship between environmentalism and veganism.

Social Justice: Advocate for food sovereignty, environmental justice, and human rights while acknowledging the intersectionality of these issues. Encourage programs aimed at resolving structural injustices and advancing a society that is more just and equal for all living things.

Beyond just eating veganism, you can live a more ethical, ecological, and compassionate existence by bringing veganism into many aspects of your everyday life. Every choice you make, whether it's to support ethical fashion labels, choose personal care products free of cruelty, or speak out in favor of environmental conservation and animal rights, can have a beneficial effect.

Exercise and Physical Activity

Exercise and physical activity are vital parts of a healthy lifestyle, whether one is vegan or not. Here are some tips for adding exercise to your vegan daily routine:

1. Select Pleasure-Seeking Activities:

Find Your Passion: Try out a variety of physical pursuits to see what you enjoy the most, including walking, jogging, cycling, swimming, dance, yoga, Pilates, weightlifting, and team sports.

Mix It Up: Add a variety of aerobic, strength training, flexibility, and balancing activities to your routines to make them engaging and exciting. This keeps you from becoming bored and works various muscle areas to improve your overall fitness.

2. Establish sensible objectives:

Start Slow: If you've never exercised before or are returning to it after a break, begin with low-intensity activities. As your fitness improves, progressively increase the duration and intensity of your workouts.

Make sure your fitness objectives are Time-bound, Specific, Measurable, Achievable, and Relevant (SMART). Whether your objective is to improve flexibility, build muscle, or run a 5K, having specific goals can help you stay motivated and focused.

3. Plan Frequent Exercises:

Make It a Habit: Just like you would with any other appointment, set aside time each day or week for exercise. Maintaining consistency is essential for making growth and benefiting from physical activity.

Be Adaptable: Since life is unpredictable, adapt your exercise routine as well. Don't be too hard on yourself if you skip a session; simply pick up where you left off the next day.

4. Remain Inspired:

Discover Your Why: Determine the reasons behind your desire to be active, such as enhancing your mood, controlling your stress, enhancing your health, or reaching particular physical objectives. When you start to lose motivation, remind yourself of these reasons.

Track Your Progress: Use a fitness journal, app, or wearable gadget to keep track of your workouts, advancement, and accomplishments. Realizing how far you've come can be very gratifying and inspiring.

5. Energize Your Exercise:

Eat Balanced Meals: Make sure you're providing your body with wholesome foods to help you with your exercise. To boost muscle recovery and supply energy, eat a well-balanced diet full of fruits, vegetables, legumes, nuts, seeds, and plant-based protein sources.

Keep Hydrated: To stay hydrated and replenish fluids lost through perspiration, drink lots of water prior to, during, and after exercise.

6. Pay Attention to Your Body:

Pay Attention to Signs: Pay attention to your body's signals of exhaustion, pain, or discomfort. When rest days are required, take them; don't ignore pain or damage.

Practice Self-Care: To aid in healing and lower stress, include restorative exercises like foam rolling, stretching, massage, and meditation in your daily schedule.

7. Maintain Contact:

Find Support: Surround yourself with people who share your passion to health and fitness, whether they be friends, family, or fellow exercise enthusiasts. Taking part in an online forum, group exercise program, or fitness class can also offer encouragement and accountability.

Celebrate Your Successes: Recognize and celebrate your accomplishments, no matter how modest, and the strides you've achieved toward your fitness objectives. Maintaining motivation and momentum can be aided by positive reinforcement.

You can enhance your general health, fitness, and well-being by prioritizing and incorporating regular physical activity into your vegan lifestyle. Always remember to engage in things you enjoy, make reasonable goals, maintain consistency, feed your body wholesome meals, pay attention to your body, and maintain relationships with encouraging groups of people. You may succeed as a vegan athlete and reach your fitness goals with commitment and persistence.

Any fitness journey, including veganism, must include tracking results and making modifications. Here's how to keep an eye on your development and make the required corrections:

1. Monitor Your Development:

Measure Key data: Keep track of relevant data such as weight, body measurements, body fat percentage, strength growth, endurance improvements, and workout performance. Use a notebook, spreadsheet, or fitness app to document your progress.

Assess Fitness Levels: Regularly assess your fitness levels by performing fitness tests or benchmarks related to your goals. Timed runs, strength and flexibility tests, and endurance trials are a few examples of this.

Document Changes: Take progress photos or keep a fitness diary to graphically document changes in your physique, energy levels, mood, and overall well-being over time.

2. Pay Attention to Your Body:

Pay Attention to Feedback: Listen to your body's messages and pay attention to how you feel during and after workouts. Note any indicators of exhaustion, soreness, pain, or discomfort, and alter your workout accordingly.

Monitor Recovery: Monitor your recovery between workouts by analyzing characteristics such as muscular discomfort, sleep quality, hunger, and energy levels. Adequate rest and recuperation are vital for minimizing burnout and injury.

3. Evaluate Nutrition:

Analyze Nutritional Intake: Make sure you're getting enough calories and macronutrients for your exercise level and objectives by assessing your nutritional intake. Use apps for tracking your food intake or speak with a qualified dietitian to evaluate your diet and make any necessary changes.

Think About Supplements: Assess if your diet is sufficient to meet your micronutrient requirements or if you may need to take supplements. Iron, calcium, omega-3 fatty acids, vitamin B12, and vitamin D are common supplements for vegans.

4. Establish New Objectives:

Reassess Objectives: Review your fitness objectives on a regular basis and make necessary adjustments in light of your development, shifting priorities, and new interests. To keep oneself motivated and focused, set new, difficult but attainable goals.

Diversify Your Training: Try different exercises, methods, or activities to provide variation to your regimen. This encourages general fitness and skill development while warding off boredom, plateaus, and overuse issues.

5. Seek Advice and Assistance:

Seek Professional Advice: Based on your requirements and goals, fitness specialists such as personal trainers, coaches, or exercise physiologists can offer individualized direction and support.

Join Communities: For accountability, support, and encouragement, get in touch with like-minded people via social media groups, online forums, or fitness communities. Ask questions, discuss your progress, and gain knowledge from others' experiences.

6. Remain Steady:

Keep Up the Consistency: Even when progress seems to be stalling or slowing down, keep up the consistency of your exercises, diet, and recuperation routines. Sustainable outcomes and long-term success require consistency throughout time.

Celebrate Your Milestones: Whether you're setting a new personal record, learning a new skill, or accomplishing a fitness-related objective, acknowledge and celebrate your accomplishments along the road. Acknowledge your accomplishments and make use of them as inspiration to keep going.

You may make educated changes to your workout regimen and keep moving closer to your health and fitness objectives as a vegan by keeping a close eye on your progress, listening to your body, assessing your nutrition, setting new goals, getting support, and being consistent. Recall that growth requires perseverance, patience, and commitment; thus, have faith in the process and relish the voyage.

Summary

In summary, living a vegan lifestyle entails more than just dietary decisions; it also entails a comprehensive approach to ethics, environmental sustainability, and health. Adopting veganism entails a compassionate way of living that advances the welfare of animals, the environment, and the self.

We have covered a wide range of topics related to veganism in this guide, such as advantages, difficulties, and useful advice for applying vegan concepts to diverse spheres of life. Veganism offers a diverse range of lifestyle choices that are in line with one's beliefs and ideals, from plant-based diet and ethical consumption to exercise and environmental advocacy.

As we've covered, adopting a vegan lifestyle calls for commitment, knowledge, and an openness to trying out novel meals, goods, and habits. People can positively impact both their own lives and the world around them by adopting mindful decisions that align with vegan beliefs.

veganism is a compassionate, sustainable, and empowered way of life that has the ability to improve the health and well-being of all living things. It is not simply a diet. Adopting a vegan lifestyle offers a route towards increased fulfillment, compassion, and well-being, regardless of your motivations—animal welfare, environmental issues, or personal health objectives.

As you proceed on your vegan journey, keep yourself updated, stay involved in encouraging communities, and be receptive to new experiences and education. Together, we can

make the world a more compassionate place for
people, animals, and the environment.

THE END